Because We Care

This book is dedicated to Montefiore and the remarkable clinical and research team working together to understand the biology of Alzheimer and related Dementias. It is through this unique and innovative research which will one day provide more effective therapies than the treatments currently available.

Ruth Swerdloff Clinical Research Fund at Montefiore

A special thank you to Dr. Mark Mehler and Tracey Dupree for making this all possible.

Library of Congress Control Number:		2011904596
ISBN:	Hardcover	978-1-4568-9131-2
	Softcover	978-1-4568-9130-5
	Ebook	978-1-4568-9132-9

This is an original book and guide for caregivers, volunteers and nurses and aides to use as resource when working with patients with Alzheimer's, dementia or any illness that involves memory loss. The author is not a doctor nor is she dispensing any medical advice. This guide has been created to help anyone who is a caregiver or is thinking of volunteering in a medical or hospital facility.

This book was printed in the United States of America.

To order additional copies of this book, contact:
Xlibris Corporation
1-888-795-4274
www.Xlibris.com
Orders@Xlibris.com
96511

Caring For Family Members and Patients That Need Us

Because We Care

What Families Need to Know About:

Caregivers/Volunteers

Traumatic Brain Injury

Eldercare Abuse

Fran Lewis

Contents

Part One: Caregivers

Why You Are So Special

Caregivers: What You Need To Know

By Fran Lewis

In August of 2003 my family's life drastically changed. On August 25 of that year, my mom got sick. She woke up with a sharp pain in her back and could hardly breathe. She called my Aunt Tova and told her to come down to her apartment and not to call my sister or me. She wanted to handle this without worrying either one of us. However, this was not to be.

My Aunt Tova called 911 and they responded to the call but insisted that one of her children be present when they did the initial exam and assessment. I was and still am the only one who knows what meds my mom takes and how often and the proper dosage.

After dealing with the preliminary issues and arriving at the hospital, the staff immediately addressed my mother's issues and concerns. They did numerous tests to find out what had caused her problem. From what she was saying, it sounded like she did not remember taking her blood thinner medicine and had overdosed on it by accident. She had always been very careful with her Coumadin. However, she had been forgetting to take it and was forgetting a lot more too. Frightening as this might seem it only got worse.

From this hospital, she was taken by ambulance to another one where they thought they could address what they believed was an aortic aneurysm. However, this was incorrect.

The following morning I received a call from the heart surgeon in charge of my mom's case asking permission to operate before it was too late. Of course, I did not hesitate and allowed him to save her life. Fortunately, I got there just in time to see her before surgery. This was the last time she would sound lucid or clear for a very long time. She came out of the operation with many more problems. She had died twice on the table and had to be revived. (I was told this later on) She began to slur her words and not understand what was happening around her. The physical operation was a success but her mental capacity for dealing with things and understanding what was happening around her greatly diminished.

When she finally came home from the hospital 2 weeks later she had to reenter the next day due to complications that no one realized when she was discharged. Because of four more stays in the hospital my family and I noticed that her ability to process information and deal with daily situations had been compromised by the surgery and the anesthesia that was given. She herself realized that she could not remain alone for any long period.

Due to all of the stays in the hospital and many other factors that changed her ability to care for herself, we were forced to find help for her by enlisting VNS to find us aides to care for her the right way. Unfortunately, this turned out to be costly to my family and me. I had to change my lifestyle and my way of living. I had to retire from teaching early and find other interests that I could pursue at home. One of course is writing books and the other short stories is a great outlet. I have even tried to publicize the fact that I am writing a book about Alzheimer's as a resource for other families to be able to learn more about this illness and to get the help and care they need for a loved one.

The only problem is that no one realizes that as the person who has to deal with nurses, doctors, home care agencies and home care providers that you still need to take time for yourself and have some kind of life. I have been nowhere for the last 7 years since my mom was diagnosed with this awful illness. She is getting much worse and now rather than make her presence known she just sits and stares all day while sitting on her chair in front of her television. She could speak in complete sentences.

Although the aides do try and sometimes succeed in taking her out in her wheelchair to get some air and possibly run into an old friend who might stop and say hello, she often rebels and refuses to leave her chair. It seems like it is her safety net and she is afraid of anything that is different.

It is really hard to remain calm and neutral when it comes to other family members that go away on vacation and do not check and see how my mom is or if there is something that I might have planned or need to do. They usually plan their flights, or trips and tell me about them when they have their trips finalized. This gets me quite upset and I often get into it with the other person. I try to explain that there are times that I would like to just do something during the day or even stay over in a hotel with my husband for the night. The home health aides are not allowed to give my mom her meds. I have to give them to her twice a day.

People forget that caregivers might actually do other things during the day. So, when I state that I am busy writing an article for a magazine, or just for one of my books, or to post on one of the many sites that I belong to, people often say, "What are you busy with, you don't work." I work from home and probably get more done in a day then they do working in an office. I never put anyone down and I respect whatever other's do. I worked for over 36 years in the NYC Public Schools and I miss working with the students in reading and writing everyday. I had fun teaching my writing classes and working with students in reading and teaching the classics was not only fun but also, rewarding.

Caregivers are people too and not just people who provide time and care for a person that is ill. They need to understand that the caregiver needs time to regroup and regenerate him or herself and take time to feel

Caregivers: Are Special People: Tips to Help You Survive

As the primary and only caregiver for my mom who has Alzheimer's I have had to develop different ways to keep myself active and my mind stimulated. All too often as a caregiver you become so immersed in taking care of the needs of the person who is ill that we forget about our own. When you make the decision to care for a family member at home you are really taking on a challenge of herculean proportion. Everyday is different and every challenge unique and must be handled differently but with kindness and care.

When a person has Alzheimer's the hardest thing to deal with is their changing and erratic behaviors. They can be calm one minute and out of control or violent the next. These behaviors tend to put a lot of stress and strain on the caregiver. Here are some ways that I found work with my mom and might help others deal with these behaviors:

Discussions and Tips

a. I find that speaking slowly and softly in a calm voice does help to calm the person down.
b. Speaking in simple sentences and short phrases does help.
c. Repeating something in different ways sometimes helps her to understand what she needs to do: It is a simple as saying Open or Open your mouth instead of eat this or trying to explain to her that she needs to eat.
d. I always call her by her first name or of course Mom to get her attention: at this point she still knows who she

is when you call her. She does not always say her name or respond verbally when asked who she is.

e. Always be positive and smile at the person. Do not let them think that you are angry with them. They are not at fault and cannot control or help their behaviors.

Cleaning and Dressing The Person

1. The one thing that is hard when trying to keep a person with this illness clean is trying to bathe the person. Fortunately, I do have four home health aides that are great. But, they often ask me to assist them when she is hard to handle. They told me they have daily schedule for bathing the person, feeding her and getting her dressed.

2. Always be kind and gentle when bathing the person and always pick out clothing that is easy to put on and easy to get off.

3. Explain, which they do, what you are going to do and why even if the person does not fully understand.

4. They always make sure that they have the soap, sponges and the showerhead ready when bathing her. She sits on a bench in the tub, which makes it safer and prevents her from falling. She has a railing up on the side so she cannot get out by herself.

5. If a shower is not possible using a handheld showerhead, then a sponge bath might be the next best option.

6. Dressing the person is often more difficult. You need to get the person dressed at the same time each day. The one thing that I know that is important is that the person, whether they are going out or not, should get dressed everyday. They need to have their hair and nails groomed and cleaned and look as normal as possible.

7. If the person with AD is still able to choose what they want to wear, then let them have the choice. It will

make them feel better and show that they are being treated with respect and dignity.

8.   I find that elastic waists in pants are easier for the aides to dress her.

9.   Slip on shoes are the easier than tying knots in sneakers or walking shoes.

Eating: this can be a real challenge especially in the late stages of the illness. Here are some tips to making that easier for you as the caregiver.

1.   If the person is having trouble chewing certain foods or if the foods are hard to swallow, you can puree the foods in a blender turning it into a softer consistency to be eaten. I find that when the aides make chicken soup and add pasta, potatoes, and other vegetables it is easier for my mom to eat the soup if it is pureed in a blender.

2.   If the person is aware of what they might want to eat you might give that person some choices as to what they might want. I would limit the choices to 2 so as not to overwhelm the person with too much decision-making.

3.   You need to choose foods that allow the person to eat independently and hopefully without having to be fed or needing too much assistance.

4.   The one thing that is vital is that since the amount of foods or food the person consumes will eventually decrease as the disease does progress, you need to make sure that they drink a lot of fluids to prevent dehydration.

5.   It is necessary to make sure that there is nothing in the foods that is difficult to swallow because as the disease does progress it will become harder for the person to swallow and you need to avoid them choking.

Incontinence: You need to make sure that the nurse assigned to your parent's case or the person who are the caregiver for knows which Home Care Agency will provide the supplies needed on a monthly basis rather than having you pay for them out of pocket. You need to follow these tips too:

1.   Set up a daily schedule for the person to go to the bathroom. The aides change my mom every 2 hours to prevent rashes, sores and chafing. They make sure that they have A&D ointment on hand as well as Destin or BalmX in order to make sure that she does not get any sores of any kind.

2.   If the person starts to fidget and gets restless that can often be sign that the person should be taken to the bathroom on the spot. (If they are still capable of using the bathroom.)

3.   Be aware that accidents will happen and you need to stay calm and be understanding. The first time this happened to my mom she was in the hospital and did realize that she was forgetting to go to the bathroom. She often rang for the nurse who never came. I think part of her problem came because she just didn't get there in time and the poor staffing on her floor of people that did not really concern themselves with patients that are incontinent. I know that they do get busy and backed up but it became apparent that this was going to be an issue. She did not want to wear the diapers and wanted to use the bedpan or the commode.

4.   To prevent nighttime accidents, limit the amount of fluids the person drinks before going to bed.

5.   If the person is aware of whether they need to use the bathroom and you are going on a long trip you might want to learn where the rest stops are located on your route so you can stop. Have the person take extra clothes

in case of an accident. I know that with my mom we made sure that she had a depend or pull up diaper on top of her underwear to prevent this issue from causing her any embarrassment.

Sleeping and Wandering

1. My mom does not sleep throughout the night. When we first found out she had the illness she even tried to leave the apartment and go shopping in the middle of the night. She left one morning and walked to the bakery to get bread. Not really knowing where and why she did that, she stopped a stranger in a car to drive her home. Lucky for her the person knew her. When I got the call from the aide that was late in coming to care for her that she was missing and finally found, I realized that we needed more help and more hours too.

2. Make sure that you enroll the person in the Safe Return Program from the Alzheimer's Association. This is a program that helps you register the person with the necessary information needed to contact you in case the person gets lost. You receive 2 bracelets and a necklace plus labels. You can sew the labels into the clothing of the person and you can wear one bracelet and the person the other in case of an emergency both parties can be helped and contacted.

3. Keep a photo of the person in your wallet and on a table in your living room and in their home in case the person is lost and ID needs to be made by the police.

4. Keep a list of the person's medications and other vital information handy including how much medication and how often the pills are taken. Post on the refrigerator along with their plan of care if you have home care.

5. Make sure that you put sharp objects out of their reach. Unplug toaster ovens and microwaves because they might forget to turn them off when they try to use them. Prepare meals for them and leave them in the refrigerator to be warmed by you or an aide. Make sure that the locks on the front door are too high for the person to open. Make sure if there is a back door that it is secured and locked and cannot be opened. You might want to have a keyed deadbolt or an additional lock that is too high for the person to reach placed on the front door of a house or an apartment. You might even add a chain.

6. These people get disoriented and cannot tell the difference between day and night. Assure them that they are in a safe place and safe environment. Never yell at them, scold them or make them feel like they did something wrong. Remember: It is the disease NOT THEM! Causing these behaviors.

7. As the disease gets worse the person might begin seeing things, hearing things and have delusions. Hallucinations are when the person sees, hears, smells and feels that something or someone is there but it really is not.

8. Delusions are beliefs that are false from which the person is so totally convinced that something is happening and they cannot be dissuaded.

Never yell at the person and assure them that you are taking care of and getting rid of whatever is upsetting them. I remember my Aunt Tova was given Haldol in the hospital and thought she saw squirrels on the ceiling of her room and thought that she left old bread and cheese in her freezer. She made my cousin call me and I told her that I would get rid of the bread and cheese and am right there to take care of the squirrels. She even told me she saw my Uncle Irving and my father Doc who have been gone a long time.

YOU COUNT TOO!

Remember to make time for yourself and your family. Do not neglect your personal appearance or your personal needs. Make sure that you take time for yourself every day. Make sure that you develop an interest or a hobby and set aside time, as I do each time to pursue what makes you happy.

Make sure that when you feel stressed that you take a break and go out for a walk, rest or just read a book. You cannot be on 24 hours a day. Make sure that if the person needs an aide that you get the services needed in order to help you have some kind of life and time with your family.

I know that there is always one person in a family that gets the burden of the care. That of course is not right and not fair. However, you need to make sure that you get to go away even overnight or on a weekend in order to rejuvenate yourself and feel better. You deserve it. I know I need time off from giving my mom her meds every morning and every night. I sometimes feel like I am wearing a straight jacket that needs to be loosened. I wish that I could go away for a week but I know that is not in the cards. No one wants the responsibility of dealing with the agencies and the meds and the aides. It gets tough.

But, as I have been told so many times, you are doing the right thing and someday you will be blessed and rewarded. I know that I can look myself in the mirror and know that I have nothing to be guilty about and know that I am trying my best to keep my mom at home. I know that a person with AD has a limited life style. I promised her that I would never put her in a facility of any kind and I will not break that promise.

How do you know that you need to Get Help For A Loved One?

When my mom went shopping by herself to the bakery one morning and asked a total stranger to drive her home, I knew things were taking a downward slide. Asking her why she would accept a ride with someone she did not know, she looked at me and said, "I have no idea what you are talking about. That lady is my friend." She was a friend whose name she did not know nor did I.

When my mom began to exhibit the following behaviors my brother, sister and I realized we needed to get her more help than the three of us could provide. This is where you need to do research and a lot of legwork to make sure that you get the right help for your parent or loved one.

1. When someone is unable to remember things
2. Asking or repeating the same question or story multiple times
3. Lost in familiar places
4. Being unable to follow and understand directions
5. Getting disoriented about time, people and places
6. Neglecting personal safety, hygiene and nutrition
7. As in my mom's case asking a stranger for a ride home
8. Wandering the neighborhood and not remembering their own address
9. Forgetting names and places
10. As in my mom's case taking her meds more than the required number of times a day

Kindness Tips for Volunteers

1. Always say good morning when entering a patient's room
2. Address the patient by name and tell the patient your name
3. SMILE!
4. Explain the task you are going to perform before you do it and explain the task as you are performing. Patients are often leery or afraid of strangers and need to feel confident and safe with you.
5. If a patient needs assistance bathing, eating or walking help them and do not leave them before they complete the task.
6. Patients that need help eating: You need to make sure that person eats and is fed. Make sure that you do not leave the tray untouched and if you have to feed the patient you need to do it with kindness and patience.
7. Ask the patient if they need help dressing or assistance going to breakfast or any other area of the home or hospital
8. If you are bringing magazines or books allow the person to choose
9. Never speak to a patient as if they were a small child
10. Speak to people with respect and as an adult
11. Making sure that the person's environment is safe
12. Make sure you have a list of things that need to be done for that person and complete them
13. Meet with other volunteers and discuss their successes
14. When you speak to a patient make sure that you make eye contact and have their attention
15. Speak at eye level and speak clearly
16. Use simple and direct statements
17. Never raise your voice

18. Include the person in your conversation: Talk to the person not at the person
19. Never speak to them as if they are a third party and not in the same room
20. Speak to them as an adult not a small child
21. Listen to their concerns and show a lot of understanding
22. Never leave a patient in distress

Your Role Is Important and Valuable

There are many jobs that are special and important. Never think that because you are not getting paid to be a volunteer that it hinders your value, importance or role. Many of the people you come in contact with have no family members visiting, are afraid to be alone and might look forward to your visit, no matter how long or short, as the highlight of their day.

Just walking into their room and knowing that you are there to speak to them, perform a needed task or just sit and talk with can be the difference between someone giving up on life and feeling needed and special.

Everything you do has value and a purpose. Never allow anyone to tell you that you do not have be work or volunteer on a specific day because it does not matter since you are not getting paid. Work ethics need to be adhered to. Volunteer positions can lead to paying ones. You never know. Your time is valuable and what you are doing to help someone that is in these facilities is worth more than all the money in the world. Never sell what you are doing short.

Remember:

1. Remember to be sensitive to the needs of the person.
2. Understand that the diagnosis is upsetting and show compassion.
3. Remember to speak to the person as an adult and a human being and not a small child.
4. Communicate with the Alzheimer's patient
5. Have an upbeat and positive attitude
6. Understand and learn how to handle behavior changes.
7. Expect that the patient will have memory loss and over time even more.
8. Get support for yourself and make sure that you do not neglect you.
9. Speak in short, familiar words, phrases and simple sentences. Repeat yourself if necessary. Stay calm
10. Allow the person plenty of time to answer. If the person does not respond or answer reword the question.
11. Ask only one question at a time.
12. Never give negative instructions: Do not say don't or Never or you better not: Say Let's try this or Let's go over here.

We are in this together!

Working together and helping them understand

Mobility is important and your assistance makes a big difference

Shopping can help them stay focused and feeling useful!

Your visit and care makes all the difference!

Helping someone with a smile makes a difference in the other person's life.

Remember: Everything you do matters and is Special

CAREGIVERS ARE SPECIAL AND UNIQUE!

Alzheimer's Disease Ten warning signs of the disease this information comes from www.medicine.net.com

The Alzheimer's Association has developed the following list of warning signs that include common symptoms of Alzheimer's disease. Individuals who exhibit several of these symptoms would see a physician for a complete evaluation:

1. Memory loss
2. Difficulty performing familiar tasks
3. Problems with language
4. Disorientation to time and place
5. Misplacing things
6. Problems with abstract thinking
7. Misplacing things
8. Changes in mood or behavior
9. Changes in personality
10. Loss of initiative

It is normal for certain kinds of memory, such as the ability to remember lists of words, to decline with normal aging. In fact, normal individuals 50 years of age will recall only about 60% as many times on some kinds of memory tests as individuals 20 years of age. Every 20 year old is well aware of multiple times he or she could not think of an answer on a test that he or she once knew. But, most 20 year olds do not worry about forgetting something or that he or she has the early stages of Alzheimer's. But, a person 50 or 60 years of age with a few memory lapses may worry that they have the early stages of the disease.

Remembering things: However, serious memory loss, confusion and other major changes in the way our minds work are not a normal part of aging.

There are many conditions that disrupt memory and mental function. These symptoms may improve when the underlying cause is treated.

Possible reasons or causes for memory loss:

Depression Medication side effects, Excess use of alcohol, Thyroid problems, Poor diet Vitamin deficiencies, and certain infections as well as Alzheimer's disease and related dementias can cause memory loss.

What is the difference between someone with Alzheimer's and someone with normal age related memory changes.

If you experience significant memory problems you need to see a doctor. Early diagnosis and intervention methods are improving and treatment options and sources of support can improve your quality of life.

Someone with Alzheimer's

Forgets whole experiences
Rarely remembers later
Is gradually unable to follow written/spoken directions
Is gradually unable to use notes is gradually unable to care for self
Someone with normal age-related memory changes
Forgets part of an experience Often remembers later
Is usually able to follow written/-spoken directions
Is usually able to use notes is usually able to care for self

These are 10 signs of Alzheimer's disease

1. Memory loss: You forget recently learned information: this is a mot common early sign of dementia. You begin to forget more often and are unable to recall information later.
2. Difficulty performing familiar tasks:
    People with dementia often find it hard to plan or finish everyday tasks. These people may lose track of the steps involved in preparing a meal, placing a phone call or playing a game.
3. Problems with Language:
    People with Alzheimer's disease often forget simple words or substitute unusual words, making their speech or writing hard to understand. They may be unable to find the toothbrush, and may ask for that thing for my mouth instead.

4. Disorientation to time and place:
    People with this disease can become lost in their own neighborhoods, forget where they are and how they got there, and not know how to get back home.

5. Poor or decreased judgment:
    People with the disease often dress inappropriately, wearing many layers on a warm day and or little clothing in the cold. They may show poor judgment about money by giving away large amount to telemarketers over the phone.

6. Problems with abstract thinking:
    Some with Alzheimer's disease may have unusual trouble performing complex mental tasks, like forgetting what numbers are and how they should be used.

7. Misplacing things:
    A person with this disease may put things in unusual places. This person might put an iron in the freezer or a wristwatch in the refrigerator.

8. Changes in mood or behavior:
    Someone with this disease may show rapid mood swings from calm to tears to anger for no apparent reason.

9. Changes in Personality
    The personalities of people with dementia can change dramatically. They may become extremely confused, suspicious, fearful or dependent on a family member.

10. Loss of initiative:
    A person with this disease may become very passive, sitting in front of the TV for hours, sleeping more than usual or not wanted to do usual activities.

What is normal?

1. Forgetting names or appointments occasionally
2. Occasionally forgetting why you came into a room or what you planned to do
3. Sometimes having trouble finding the right word
4. Forgetting the day of the week or where you were going
5. Making questionable or debatable decision from time to time
6. Challenging to balance a checkbook
7. Misplacing keys or a wallet temporarily
8. Occasionally feeling sad or moody
9. People's personalities do change somewhat with age
10. Sometimes feeling weary of work or social obligations.

Doctor Discussion Guide

When your family member is concerned about the changes mentioned in the previous section that might indicate mild to moderate Alzheimer's disease of dementia.

The following information comes from the website of Novartis These are the questions that you need to ask your doctor:

1. Do the symptoms indicate a problem?
2. Is Alzheimer's disease dementia one of the possible things that might be causing these symptoms?
3. Are there other conditions that might be causing these symptoms?
4. Will tests be needed in order for you to make this diagnosis? Which ones?
5. How long will it be before I will know the diagnosis?
6. If it is Alzheimer's disease, what should I expect?
7. What medicines are available?

8. Can these medicines help slow the worsening of symptoms? Which ones?
9. How do these medicines work?

These are questions your doctor might ask you or a family member:

1. Are you or someone you care for?
    a. Forgetting conversations, appointments, or holidays?
    b. Having difficulty finding the right words to express their thoughts or your thoughts
    c. Repeating stories or questions
    d. Getting lost in places familiar to you

Have you or someone you care for:

    a. Forgotten how to do familiar activities, like cooking or repairing things
    b. Had difficulty doing bills of balancing the checkbook or thrown away a bill before paying it.
    c. Been misplacing things more often than usual.

Have you or someone you care for:

    a. Lost interest in friends, hobbies, or other activities that were once enjoyable
    b. Been resisting change or new activities
    c. Become more upset or angrier than usual
    d. Often felt sad.

People with memory loss or other possible warning signs of Alzheimer's may find to recognize that they have a problem and might resist following up on their symptoms. Signs of dementia may be more obvious to friends and family. The first step is to find a doctor you feel comfortable with. You local Alzheimer's Association can assist you with finding a doctor.

There is no one type of doctor that specializes in diagnosing and treating this disease. Many people usually contact their primary care doctor about their concerns. Primary care doctors often oversee the diagnostic process themselves.

Another problem people face when diagnosed with this disease is how the doctor or medical profession explains the illness and how the person is told. It heartbreaking enough for anyone to be told that this is happening to them and that your future is no longer in your control. The Alzheimer's Association suggested this to ease the way for the person and family to understand what is going to happen and to give the person a dignified diagnosis.

1. Speak directly to the person with dementia. That is the person that needs to know and understand the information.
2. Tell the truth: Doctors do not always have all of the answers but they should be honest about what they do know and why they believe the knowledge they have is the truth.
3. Test early: The patient needs an accurate diagnosis as fast as possible which gives them more time to deal and live to their fullest potential. It gives the person time to get more information about the appropriate clinical trials.
4. Take the patient's concerns seriously, regardless of their age. Age may be the biggest risk factor for this disease. It is definitely not a normal part of aging. Do not make the patient feel that their concerns are unfounded or they are old so they do not understand what is happening

to them. This disease can hit people in there 40's, 50's and 60's.

5. Deliver the news in plain but sensitive language. This is probably one of the most vital and important things that the patient needs to hear. Using language that the person can understand and is sensitive will help the person feel better and that the health care provider is showing compassion for his/her feelings

6. Coordinate with other care providers:
If the patient is seeing more than one specialist it is important that the doctors coordinate their information so that any changes in the patient can be identified early on and that they do not have to retake or repeat any tests unnecessarily.

7. Explain the purpose of different tests and what you hope to learn from them:
These tests can be both physically and emotionally draining. It helps the patient to understand the purpose of all of the tests and the duration of each test and would you hope to learn from them. There should be an option for the patient to take a breather or a break between tests that are longer in order to ask questions.

8. What tools are there that you can give the patient in order to cope and live with this disease?
Do not give the patient this diagnosis and leave them alone to deal with it. The person needs to understand what is going to happen to them they need to know if there are any medical options and what support services are available for them and their family members.

9. Work with the patient on a plan for healthy living.
Medication may help modify some of the neurological symptoms. Patients are interested in other recommendations for keeping health—like diet, exercise and social engagements.

10. Recognize that the patient is an individual and will experience the disease in his/her own or unique way. This disease affects each person in different ways and at a different rate. Telling the patient the rate that this illness will affect him/her and how fast things will go downhill needs to be addressed to that patient and not to others in general.

11. Alzheimer's is a journey, not a destination
    There is no prescription to cure this illness and doctors need to be their patient's advocate and work with them to get quality care and try to have some type of life while going through these changes.

Stages of Alzheimer's Disease

Experts have documented common patterns of symptom progression that occur in many individuals with Alzheimer's disease and developed several methods of "staging" based on these patterns. Progression of symptoms corresponds in a general way to the underlying nerve cell degeneration that takes place in Alzheimer's disease.

Nerve cell damage typically begins with cells involved in learning and memory and gradually spreads to cells that control other aspects of thinking, judgment and behavior. The damage eventually affects cells that control and coordinate movement.

Staging systems provide useful frames of reference for understanding how the disease may unfold and for making future plans. But it is important to note that all stages are artificial benchmarks in a continuous process that can vary greatly from one person to another. Not everyone will experience every symptom and symptoms may occur at different times in different individuals. People with Alzheimer's die an average of four to six years after diagnosis, but the duration of the disease can vary from three to 20 years.

The framework for this fact sheet is a system that outlines key symptoms characterizing seven stages ranging from unimpaired function to very severe cognitive decline. This framework is based on a system developed by Barry Reisberg, M.D., Clinical Director of the New York University School of Medicine's Silberstein Aging and Dementia Research Center.

Within this framework, we have noted which stages correspond to the widely used concepts of mild, moderate, moderately severe and severe Alzheimer's disease. We have also noted which stages fall within the more general divisions of early-stage, mid-stage and late-stage categories.

Stage 1: No cognitive impairment

Unimpaired individuals experience no memory problems and none are evident to a health care professional during a medical interview.

Stage 2: Very mild decline

Individuals at this stage feel as if they have memory lapses, forgetting familiar words or names or the location of keys, eyeglasses or other everyday objects. But these problems are not evident during a medical examination or apparent to friends, family or co-workers.

Stage 3: Mild cognitive decline

Early-stage Alzheimer's can be diagnosed in some, but not all, individuals with these symptoms

Friends, family or co-workers begin to notice deficiencies. Problems with memory or concentration may be measurable in clinical testing or discernible during a detailed medical interview. Common difficulties include:

- Word, or name-finding problems noticeable to family or close associates
- Decreased ability to remember names when introduced to new people
- Performance issues in social and work settings noticeable to others
- Reading a passage and retaining little material

- Losing or misplacing a valuable object
- Decline in ability to plan or organize

Stage 4: Moderate cognitive decline (Mild or early-stage Alzheimer's disease)

At this stage, a careful medical interview detects clear-cut deficiencies in the following areas:

- Decreased knowledge of recent events
- Impaired ability to perform challenging mental arithmetic. For Example, to count backward from 100 by 7s
- Decreased capacity to perform complex tasks, such as marketing, Planning dinner for guests, or paying bills and managing finances
- Reduced memory of personal history
- The affected individual may seem subdued and withdrawn, especially in socially or mentally challenging situations

Stage 5: Moderately severe cognitive decline (Moderate or mid-stage Alzheimer's disease)

Major gaps in memory and deficits in cognitive function emerge. Some assistance with day-to-day activities becomes essential. At this stage, individuals may:

- Be unable during a medical interview to recall such important details as their current address, their telephone number, or the name of the college or high school from which they graduated
- Become confused about where they are or about the date, day of the week or season

- Have trouble with less challenging mental arithmetic; for example, counting backward from 40 by 4s or from 20 by 2s
- Need help choosing proper clothing for the season or the occasion
- Usually retain substantial knowledge about them and know Their own name and the names of their spouse or children
- usually require no assistance with eating or using the toilet

Stage 6: Severe cognitive decline (Moderately severe or mid-stage Alzheimer's disease)

Memory difficulties continue to worsen, significant personality changes may emerge, and affected individuals need extensive help with daily activities. At this stage, individuals may:

- Lose most awareness of recent experiences and events as well as of their surroundings
- Recollect their personal history imperfectly, although they generally recall their own name
- Occasionally forget the name of their spouse or primary caregiver but generally can distinguish familiar from unfamiliar faces
- Need help getting dressed properly; without supervision, may make such errors as putting pajamas over daytime clothes or shoes on wrong feet
- Experience disruption of their normal sleep/waking cycle
- Need help with handling details of toileting (flushing toilet, wiping. And disposing of tissue properly)
- Have increasing episodes of urinary or fecal incontinence
- Experience significant personality changes and behavioral symptoms, including suspiciousness and delusions (for example, believing that their caregiver is an impostor);

hallucinations (seeing or hearing things that are not really there); or compulsive, repetitive behaviors such as hand wringing or tissue shredding

- Tend to wander and become lost

Stage 7: Very severe cognitive decline (Severe or late-stage Alzheimer's disease)

This is the final stage of the disease when individuals lose the ability to respond to their environment, the ability to speak, and, ultimately, the ability to control movement.

Frequently individuals lose their capacity for recognizable speech, although words or phrases may occasionally be uttered

- Individuals need help with eating and toileting and there is general incontinence
- Individuals lose the ability to walk without assistance, then the ability to sit without support, the ability to smile, and the ability to hold their head up. Reflexes become abnormal and muscles grow rigid. Swallowing is impaired.

Here is information about support groups, services and information you might need to get the help and services you need.

1. Alzheimer's Disease Educations and Referral (ADEAR) Center P.O. Box 8250
   Silver Springs, MD 20907-8250 1-800-438-4380
   www.alzheimers.nia.nih.gov

   This service of the National Institute of Aging offers information and publications on diagnosis, treatment, patient caregiver needs, long-term care, education and training; research related to AD. Staff answer telephone, e-mail, and written requests and make referrals to local and national resources.

2.   Alzheimer's Association 225 N. Michigan Avenue, Suite 1700 Chicago, Il.60601-7633 1-800-272-3900 www.alz.org

This nonprofit association supports families and caregivers of patients with Alzheimer's disease and funds research. Chapters nationwide provide referrals to local resources and services. They sponsor support groups and educational programs.

3.   Children of Aging Parents P.O. Box 167 Richboro, P.A. 18954 1-800-227-7294 www.caps4caregivers.org

This is a nonprofit group that provides information and materials for adults caring for their older parents. Caregivers of people with this disease might find their resources and information helpful.

4.   Eldercare Locator 1-800-677-1116 www.eldercare.gov

This service of the Administration of Aging, funded by the Federal Government, provides information and referrals to respite care and other home and community services offered by State and Area Agencies on aging.

5. Family Caregiver Alliance 180 Montgomery Street Suite 1100 San Francisco, CA 94104 1-800-445-8106 www.caregiver.org

Family Caregiver Alliance is a community-based nonprofit organization offering support services for those caring for adults and AD, stroke, Traumatic Brain Injuries, and other cognitive disorders. Programs and services include an Information Clearinghouse fro FCA's publications.

Telling Others About
An Alzheimer Diagnosis

When you learn that someone you care about has Alzheimer's, you may hesitate to tell the person that he or she has the disease.

You may also have a hard time deciding whether to tell family and friends. Once you are emotionally ready to discuss the diagnosis, how will you break the news? Here are some suggestions for talking about the disease with others.

Respect the person's right to know

- You may want to protect the person by withholding information. But your loved one is an adult with the right to know the truth. It can be a relief to hear the diagnosis, especially if the person had suspected he or she had Alzheimer's disease.
- In many cases, people who are diagnosed early are able to participate in important decisions about their healthcare, legal and financial planning.
- While there is no current cure for Alzheimer's; life will not stop with the diagnosis. There are treatments and services that can make life better for everyone.
  Plan how to tell the person
- Talk with doctors, social workers and others who work with people who have Alzheimer's to plan an approach for discussing the diagnosis.
- Consider a "family conference" to tell the person about the diagnosis. He or she may not remember the discussion, but may remember that people cared enough to come together. You may need to have more than one meeting to cover the details.

- Shape the discussion to fit the person's emotional state, medical condition and ability to remember and make decisions.
- Pick the best time to talk about the diagnosis. People with Alzheimer's may be more receptive to new information at different times of the day. Don't provide too much information at once. Listen carefully to the person. They often signal the amount of information they can deal with through their question and reactions. Later, you can explain the symptoms of Alzheimer's and talk about planning for the future and getting support. Help the person accept the diagnosis the person may not understand the meaning of the diagnosis or may deny it. Accept such reactions and avoid further explanations.

If they respond well, try providing additional information. The person with Alzheimer's may forget the initial discussion but not the emotion involved. If telling them upsets them, hearing additional details may trigger the same reaction later. 1.800.272.3900 | www.alz.org

- Reassure your loved one. Express your commitment to help and give support. Let the person know that you will do all you can to keep your lives fulfilling.
- Be open to the person's need to talk about the diagnosis and his or her emotions.
- Look for nonverbal signs of sadness, anger or anxiety. Respond with love and reassurance.
- Encourage the person to join a support group for individuals with memory loss. Your local Alzheimer's Association can help you locate a group. To find an Association near you, please call 1.800.272.3900 or go to www.alz.org.

Telling family and friends

An Alzheimer diagnosis doesn't only affect the person receiving it. The lives of family members and friends may also drastically change.

- Be honest with family and friends about the person's diagnosis. Explain that Alzheimer's is a brain disease, not a psychological or emotional disorder.
- Share educational materials from the Alzheimer's Association. The more that people learn about the disease, the more comfortable they may feel around the person.
- Invite family to support groups sponsored by your local Alzheimer's Association.
- Realize that some people may drift out of your life, as they may feel uncomfortable around the person or may not want to help provide care.
- Alzheimer's disease can also impact children and teens. Just as with any family member, be honest about the person's diagnosis with the young people in your life. Encourage them to ask questions.

Websites and Research About this Illness

For your Information

www.alz.org www.medicinenet.com/alzheimers_disease/page8. htm Fisher Center for Alzheimer's www.alzinfo.org/alzheimers-treatment-overview.as;#3 www.exelonpatch.com/info/For_the_Caregiver/saftey.jsp

There are agencies that you can call to help you find the services you need.

1. Medicare
2. Medicare
3. Visiting Nurse Service will come in and evaluate the patient for services to start and then help you to get Medicaid for your friend or family member.
4. Your Local Congressman can help with some of their staff members who are trained to help you get the additional services you might need or to keep services that you already have in place.

Final Care: What You Need to Know about when the End Is Near

The most difficult stage of course of any illness if the final one leading to the passing of the loved one whether Alzheimer's or any other terminal illness twenty hour care seven days a week is apparent and needed. Caregivers need to realize that the last stage of Alzheimer's is difficult and very challenging. End of life decisions now have to be made and final arrangements should be in place. Understanding and anticipating what is to come is vital. Even with the most loving and outstanding care the end result is still the same. In this horrific last stage the patient or loved one will lack the ability to communicate directly, verbally interact, will be as my mom's aide's know, totally depended for all personal care on the home health aides, and is confined to her bed or lift chair 24/7. She no longer walks although she has use of her limbs. She cannot stand or walk even with a walker for balance. Most patients cannot recognize familiar pictures, people or objects. However, if you show my mom some really old pictures from the past at times she does remember the figures in them. Dependency on others becomes their way of life. As in my mom's case it is vital that she receives professional care from those trained and qualified to handle care for Alzheimer's patients. Although I monitor the care, administer her meds twice a day and handle all of the paperwork required by Medicare and Medicaid, and the home health care agencies, without the four aides that so brilliantly and lovingly care for her I do not know what I would do nor could I sleep at night. But, my cell phone is always on and right next to me if needed.

As a caregiver or even an aide there are four important areas that must be stressed:

1. All practical care and assistance related to dressing, feeding, bathing and the caregiver or aide must handle daily activities. Skills, task and routines need to be carefully charted-listed and recorded either on a plan of care or by the caregiver taped on the refrigerator.
2. Speaking to the patient politely, lovingly and treating the person with respect and dignity in a nurturing environment so they feel safe and secure is vital.
3. As a caregiver you are going to need help, support or aid from other family members-health agents, legal and financial advisors
4. Grief Support: after losing your loved one you might need counseling or to join a grief support group

Other Considerations:

1. Decide on whether you will keep the person at home or in a facility
2. Seek financial and legal advice while the person can participate
3. Hospice Services
4. Rabbi, priest, chaplain, clergy to speak with for support
5. Wills and living wills
6. Family Conflicts: end of life directives need to be spelling out in writing-witnessed and notarized by the patient before it is too late for them to make that vital decision
7. Bereavement support
8. Implementing decisions for or against prolonged life treatments

Resources that I used for this pamphlet:

www.alz.org
www.nia.nih.gov
www.nia.nih.gov/Alzheimers
www.nia.nih.gov/Alzheimers/Publications/caregiverguide.htm#intro
www.nia.nih.gov/Healthinformation/Publications/forgetfulness.htm

Important Resources and Information

1. What are the signs of memory loss?
2. What are the stages of the disease?
3. What can you do when you are diagnosed with it?
4. What are the changes in behaviors?
5. What safety measures can you take at home?
6. What personal care changes occur and need to be addressed?
7. Caregiver Information
8. Supporting the caregiver
9. Resources to get help and support
10. Changes in eating and sleeping

Part Two: Protecting Your Brain

Traumatic Brain Injury

WHAT YOU NEED TO KNOW AND UNDERSTAND ABOUT TRAUMATIC BRAIN INJURY AND MORE

Section Two: Traumatic Brain Injury: What you need to know and understand and Traumatic Brain Injuries and More

Traumatic Brain Injury

1. How to avoid brain injuries
2. What safety precautions should you knows about and takes?
3. How are they treated?
4. What are the permanent effects?
5. What resources are out there to help if you have a Traumatic Brain Injury?

An injury to your brain can result in loss of function and results in brain cell death. Traumatic Brain Injury is an external trauma to the head. It can also be caused by a violent movement of the head as a result of a fall, car crash or being shaken. When I was 17, I was in a serious car accident on a back road going to South Fallsburg. Till this day I cannot tell you what really happened or who was at fault. All I remember is that I was sitting the center seat in the rear of the car with my cousin and the driver's son. The driver and a friend of my mom were in the front two seats. My cousin and I sat quietly in the back of the car. We were going shopping for our mothers and were really concentrating on the scenery and not talking about anything in particular. As we rounded a corner on this back road another car was coming directly at us and the next thing I remember, which was not a lot was lights out. Someone yelled look out but I guess not fast or loud enough. It was a fatal head-on collision causing the person in the front passenger seat to die instantly and I was thrown from the back of the car through the windshield and back. The next thing I remember was sitting on a bench on a porch and having been pulled out by an unknown person. Coming out of my stupor, I looked around and did not even recognize my surroundings, or that I was severely injured. My head hurt, my memory seemed fogged, and I had no idea who the people that were sitting near me were. My cousin tried to tell me who she was and so did the son of the driver, but I just stared back at them afraid. I kept asking more questions about what happened, where we were going and who they were but nothing seemed to click. What saved me from instant death was the fall that I was wearing on my head stuffed with sanitary napkins that must have cushioned the hard blow to my head. I later found out that I suffered a severe head concussion, amnesia, blood clots and hematomas to my legs and more. There were no SEAT BELTS in the back of the car and the passenger and driver in the front were not buckled in. My mother's friend died of a broken neck: she did not have a chance. The driver of the other car had leg injuries and my cousin lost her teeth and the others had minor injuries.

Traumatic Brain Injury is serious and can have lasting results. But, car crashes are not the only causes of TBI. Bicycle accidents, sports injuries, severe falls, acts of violence, blows to the head and even gunshot wounds are causes of TBI. That is the purpose of this article to make you aware of the causes and how to prevent TBI.

Avoiding Traumatic Brain Injury requires adhering to certain safety precautions when driving, engaging in sports activities and even exercising. It is a simple as wearing a seat belt in a car whether in the passenger or driver's seat or wearing a helmet when riding a bike. Here are some important tips or suggestions that might save your life:

Everyone needs to be safety conscious. These tips are not just for children but adults too. Your head is not a rubber ball and will not bounce back into place if injured. If you fall, get hit hard or even worse get shot you might never recover. Racing cars, riding a bike, a horse, scooter, skateboard, snowboarding and skiing you need to wear a helmet. It's a simple as buckling up your seatbelt in a car, truck or van. Sitting in your seat on a bus or a train. Using booster seats and properly fitted car seats for children.

Do not get behind the wheel of any vehicle if you are drunk or have taken any type of prescription drugs that make you tired. Never drive under the influence of any other kind of drug either.

Wear helmets when participating in sports: biking, riding a motorcycle, snowmobile, all-terrain vehicles or even playing contact sports like football, soccer, boxing and hockey wear a helmet. When up at bat in a baseball game: Wear that HELMET!

Horseback riding is fun but you should wear a helmet incase of being thrown by the horse or in a riding competition.

Skiing, snowboarding: Wear that helmet!

How to Remain Safe At Home?

1.   Accidents can happen anywhere. Just because you are at home cooking in the kitchen or showering in the bathroom does not mean that something might not happen. Walking on a torn or frayed carpet or area rug, a wet mat that is not secured and has the proper rubber tips on it can cause a fall almost anywhere in your home.

2.   Step stools should have grab bars on it to reach items that are high up in cabinets

3.   Windows should have window guards with small children living there and they should be properly locked as well as terrace or patio doors that are on high floors.

4.   When vacuuming beware of the cord and make sure that your foot/legs do not become tangled as you move the machine about.

5.   Install handrails on staircases

6.   Install safety gates: top and bottom of stairs when young children are present: Keep gates locked

7.   Flames on stoves should not be left on without something cooking on it and burners should not be left unattended.

8.   Remove tripping hazards like small rugs, mats which are dangerous including welcome mats which can cause accidents too.

9.   Use non-slip mats with tabs in the bathroom

10. Grab bars should be installed in the shower or tub

11. Exercise

12. Make sure your vision is checked

13. If you have playground equipment in your backyard make sure that every safety precaution is taken and make sure you have the equipment regularly checked out.

14. Surface of the playground should be made of absorbing material like hardwood, mulch or sand

15. Make sure that swings, slides, monkey bars and other equipments are checked and that chains that keep them sturdy are properly secured and the slides are not wobbly as children go down and the handrails are secured.

Symptoms of Traumatic Brain Injury

Believe it or not statistics have proved that every 21 seconds someone in the United States sustains Traumatic Brain Injury. Americans suffer from head injuries on an annual basis and over 80,000 of these are irreversible. According to the Center for Disease Control and Prevention head injuries are the leading cause of death in young adults and children. Forty percent of all injury related deaths in the United States are head injuries. After suffering a memory loss and severe head injury in a fatal car accident I realize how important and vital it is to just simply wear a seatbelt.

These are the major symptoms to look out for when being concerned about Traumatic Brain Injury:

These are a list of symptoms to be aware of and if you exhibit any or all of this CALL THE DOCTOR OR GO TO AN ER!

In Adults:

1. Headaches or neck pain that is persistent and does not go away.
2. Trouble concentrating, or decision-making
3. Slow thinking, speaking, or reading
4. Getting lost or easily confused and not being able to follow simple directions
5. Trouble remembering names
6. Feeling tired all of the time
7. Having little or no energy or drive
8. Mood swings
9. Changes in sleep patterns-trouble sleeping or sleeping too much
10. Lightheaded or dizzy or losing your balance

11. An urge to throw up
12. Increase in your sensitivity to lights, sounds or distractions
13. Blurred vision or eyes that tired too easily
14. Ringing in the ears
15. Loss of sense of smell

Children

1. Tired or listless
2. Irritable or cranky or cannot be consoled
3. Changes in eating—will not eat or nurse
4. Changes in sleep patterns
5. Changes in the way the child plays
6. Changes in school performance
7. Loss of interest in favorite games or toys
8. Loss of interest in learning new skills
9. Loss of balance and unsteady walking
10. Vomiting

Causes of Traumatic Brain Injury

There are many causes that contribute to Traumatic Brain Injuries. Traumatic Brain Injury is serious. You need to protect your brain without it you would not be able to function, think or process information: You have only one Brain and you need to take precautions:

These are the primary causes of TBI:

1. Car accidents
2. Falls
3. Bicycle or motorcycle accidents
4. Sports related
5. Assault/ gun shot wound
6. Violence

Your brain helps you understand and interpret information and the world around you. When your brain is injured there is a disruption in its' ability to store, process and retrieve information. It can also interfere with your ability to control your emotions and interact with others.

How Do You Know?

Many times we avoid the fact that we have a problem and tend to ignore it. DON'T! As with my head injury I could not remember the incident, nor can I remember it now. I had trouble remembering the names of the people in the car the names of my family members when they came to the hospital. Several days later I found a shopping list in my bag that I wrote before we left and things started to fall into place after reading it. It is common to forget what happened before an injury occurred but symptoms cannot and should not be ignored.

How Do I Know If I Need Medical Help?

Your injuries can range from the scalp and face including lacerations, bruising or abrasions. More common symptoms are:

1. Loss of consciousness
2. Concussion
3. Brain contusion
4. Skull fracture
5. Hematoma

However, there are numerous symptoms that you need to be aware of and address if they are also present:

Headaches
Lethargy
Balance
Nausea
Fatigue
Bad taste in the mouth
Slurred speech
Neck pain
Anxiety
Irritability
Depression
Difficulty concentrating
Memory loss
Trouble collecting thoughts
Trouble sleeping
Dilated pupils
Drainage of blood or clear fluid from the nose to ears
Weakness or numbness in the limbs.

Other causes of Traumatic Brain Injury

Trucking accidents
Defective products
Unlawful alcohol sales
Slip and fall
Work place injuries

Traumatic Brain Injuries and Alzheimer's

A head trauma and its role in the development of Alzheimer's are undergoing study. Most likely a serious head injury shortens the period between Alzheimer's disease and its onset would develop. There may be a link between TBI and the onset of Alzheimer's years later. The main point to address is to address these injuries and follow the safety precautions to avoid them.

Final Points:

Seniors and Kids are prone to having the most accidents. 1.8 million seniors 65 and over are treated in the ER for falls.

Seniors: How Can they Prevent Falls:

1. Exercise regularly
2. Install grab bars and non-slip mats
3. Handrails should be installed
4. Make sure you have ample lighting
5. Be aware and careful of lose cords-extension cords: Be aware when you vacuum that you do not trip on the cord and that cords are plugged in properly in outlets.
6. Be mindful of all medications with side effects especially if you are going to drive or operate machinery.
7. Wear non-slip shoes and slippers
8. Make sure you get your vision tested

Preventing children from falling:

1. Do not leave a child alone or unattended in a tub/shower
2. Wall mounted-non-accordion safety gates should be installed
3. Install doorknob covers-locks-stops and door holders
4. Window guards should be installed
5. Never leave a side rail on a crib down—make sure it is secured and locked in place
6. Children sleeping in bunk beds-guard rails need to be placed on top bunks
7. In Cars: Car seats
8. Supermarkets; Secure child in shopping cart with seatbelt
9. Make sure in restaurants you use a highchair that the child cannot slip out from the bottom and there is something to secure them in the seat
10. Dry floors
11. Keep stairs clean

Remember these injuries can be avoided using the proper precautions.

Traumatic Brain Injury is serious and can leave lasting effects on adults, children and seniors. Take Precautions.

Characteristics of Traumatic Brain Injury

How does it impair your senses or your thinking skills?

1. Slows down your thinking
2. Makes it difficult to complete tasks and jobs
3. Hard to remember things-memory and learning is hard
4. You might have trouble concentrating
5. Your might have difficulty sequencing
6. You might disregard safety rules

7. You might have changes in your senses
8. You might have experience these behavioral changes too:
    a. Anxiety
    b. Impatience
    c. Low self-esteem
    d. Mood swings/changes
    e. Hard to cope
    f. Self-centered
    g. Headaches
    h. Constant pain
    i. Your balance might be off/walking
    j. Appetite changes
    k. Trouble swallowing
    l. Seizures
    m. Speech might be slurred
    n. No speech
    o. Bladder or bowel problems

Seek medical help if you notice marked changes
Hopefully symptoms will improve but they should not be ignored.

Resources

www.allabouttbi.com
www.cdc.gov/TraumaticBraininjury
www.cdc.gov/HomeandRecreationalsafety/Playground-Injuries/
    playgroundinjuries-factsheet.htm#pl

*http://www.michigan.gov/documents/mdch/Resources_for_Persons_*
    with_Brain_Injury_and_Their_Families_201404_7.pdf

http://www.cdc.gov/injuryresponse/index.html
http://www.braininjury.com/symptoms.html

Part Three: Protecting The Elderly

Eldercare Abuse

WHAT YOU NEED TO KNOW, UNDERSTAND AND LEARN TO PREVENT THIS ABUSE

Eldercare abuse is prevalent in nursing homes, hospitals and even at home. All too often aides, nurses and even caregivers are cruel to those that are, unable to speak for themselves and fight back. Newspapers, online sites and news commentators report these incidents on a daily basis yet the abuse continues. Imagine that the abuser is someone you know—a family member you think you can trust-spouse who is supposed to protect you or health care worker.

How Widespread or large is this problem:

If cases are not reported victims are not indentified—it is hard to state or answer this question. However, after visiting nursing homes, listening to some health care providers and touring some hospitals—it was not hard to see. In one nursing home I witnessed the head administrator push a patient away from her when she tried to give her a hug. In two other homes many of the patients were lined up in wheelchairs in the hallway either asleep, looking drugged or just staring into outer space with no one talking or interacting with them.

Elder Care Abuse: Defined:

This is no doubt that it is purposeful-intentional and cruel. Defined as the intentional or neglected acts by someone trusted by a person: Caregiver-spouse-aide-nurse-leading to harm of any elderly person who is vulnerable. Physical abuse neglect: can be emotional-psychological verbal and even financial. Exploitation-sexual abuse-abandonment are forms of neglect and abuse. In some states self-neglect is considered abuse. Dealing with home care agencies for my mom has been a real eye-opener and totally enlightening. Replacement aides are often negligent-unfeeling and in several cases abusive both verbally and physically.

One specific incident comes to mind when the regular night aide was ill and the replacement came in. The day aides explained and remained for over one hour. My mom's condition and behaviors warranted twenty-four hour care and she cannot eat, move or speak for herself. The aide explained everything to this young arrogant person before leaving. About one hour later she called and claimed my mom had thrown her walker at her. That was a real laugh. My mom was sitting in her chair and watching television with a black and blue mark on her wrist that she did not have before. My mom is fragile and cannot lift a pencil by herself. She was sitting behind the table writing down what she claimed happened and had a smirk on her face letting me know she was not telling it straight. At that point I called the agency and demanded they send another aide and that I was going to file a major complaint against her.

Elder Care Abuse shows or manifests itself in many forms:

Physical
Self-neglect
Emotional
Sexual
Financial abuse
Abandonment

How Do You Prevent Elder Abuse?

1. Report suspected mistreatment to local adult and protective agencies or police
2. Keep in contact with neighbors and friends—do not isolate person—be aware of what caregiver/aides are doing
3. Be aware of possibility of abuse—take note of elderly neighbors—change of attitude withdrawn-nervous-fearful-sad and report
4. Contact your local area agency or aging office
5. Volunteer to help in senior centers
6. Learn about Elder Abuse World Day

Resources

www.ncea.ava.gov
www.ncea-info@aoa.hhs.gov
www.ncea.aoa.gov

Nursing Home Abuse

Very prominent in the news is nursing home abuse. After visiting many homes to assess them or to visit friends of my mom and my aunt who was in hospice environment and to see just what kind of care people received. I made my own decision as my mom POA to keep her safe at home. That does not mean that I do not have to monitor her home care. It just means I am right there in case anything happens. Of course that puts the burden on me to monitor the aides, agency and homecare services. After visiting more than 15 homes and seeing some of her friends in these facilities I realized that I made the right decision. That is not to say that all nursing homes are neglectful or poorly run. It just means unless you are there on a daily basis the person might not receive the care they need. Visibility is the key! When placing a parent or loved on in these facilities you need to do your homework first. Check out their website and learn about their services. Check out any complaints filed against the home. Visit at varied unannounced times. Ask to see the patients that are the most seriously ill and need the most care. Observe how the staff interacts with these patients and listen to the tone of their voices and observe their body language.

As you walk around observe the cleanliness of the place and the people to see if they are well groomed and cared for. See how they are dressed or if too many are left to fend for themselves in their rooms because they cannot speak up or feed themselves. Observe what happens when a patient does not eat: do they feed them or are they ignored?

Every home should have a daily plan or calendar posted with the days activities. They should have copies to give visitors and family members too. What happens when a patient needs medical care not provided by the staff of the home? How fast do they call 911 for assistance? How fast do they call the family member? How are meds administered? Do they continue with the ones the patient is taking before entering the home or do they change them and if so why? Do they keep in contact with the patient's primary doctor or is that doctor no longer kept informed? With my Aunt my cousins take her to her own doctors keeping her medications and physical needs the same.

Nursing Home regulations require they participate in Medicare and Medicaid programs to conform to certain requirements for quality of care. Federal laws regulate quality of care and New York State exact care and the laws too. So—why are there so many incidents of abuse? Nursing homes must conduct an initial comprehensive evaluation of each patient and reassess periodically to see if there are any significant changes in the condition of the person. As with the home health aides and caregivers, even if they are family members, Nursing Homes are supposed to generate an individual plan of care specific for each patient that must be documented in the person's file or clinical record. There are many homes that do not provide the required care and patients deteriorate and die violating federal and state laws but then it is too late. It is even possible that the home submitted false claims to the government if they receive from Medicare and Medicaid.

Suspect Abuse Call: DON'T WAIT: TAKE ACTION

Pierro Law at 1-866-951-Plan

Eldercare Locater at 1-800-677-1116

911

To report suspected abuse in a nursing home or long-term care facility, contact your state specific agency. To find the listing visit the Long-Term Care Ombudsman website at:

http://www.Itcombudsman.org/ombudsman

Contact the National Center on Elder Care Abuse/NCEA
c/o University of Delaware
Center for Community Research and Service 297 Graham Hall
Newark, DE 19716
www.cec.gov/ViolencePrevention/DELTA/index.html

Frequently Asked Questions:
Alzheimer's

1. Is it hereditary?
2. How can I find out if I am going to have it or have the gene?
3. What causes the plague to develop in the brain?
4. What about too much anesthesia?
5. Can diet and exercise delay or prevent the onset of the illness or the illness entirely?
6. Can it ever be reversed?
7. What research is being done and what are the latest medications that are being used or tested other than Namenda and Aricept?
8. What are the major warning signs?
9. How do I know what is normal and when I should be concerned?
10. When do I need help?
11. What agencies provide the answers?
12. Where Can I learn about support groups?

These questions and any that you have of your own need to be with you when you speak to your doctor or your family member's doctor?

Plus:
Medications and how they are monitored
When to stop the person from driving and take away the keys?
When is 24 /7 care vital?

Frequently Asked Questions About
Traumatic Brain Injury

1.   How does the Kessler Foundation work with patients with Traumatic Brain Injury?

Kids, adults, infants

2.   What type of equipment is used to restore motor skills?
3.   What exercises or therapy is used to restore brain function-reading, writing-math and language skills?
4.   What type of physical therapy is done to restore movement?
5.   What about occupational therapy?
6.   What is done to restore mental brain function?
7.   What type of Traumatic Brain is most prevalent?
8.   What does the foundation do to work with these injuries and which are most successful?
9.   What besides home accidents, sports injuries or accidents in car or moving vehicle are the prime causes of TBI in teens and small children?
10.   What medical reasons or causes might attribute to result in TBI?

If a person has a Stroke or massive Heart Attack and falls on a hard floor-hitting their heads square on their face would that result in TBI and what kind and how severe?

When someone loses oxygen to the brain for more than 27 minutes and their lower brain function is still there:

1. In a small child could the higher function be restored
2. Infants
3. Adults

When is it too late? What If someone tries to administer CPR and has no idea how chest compressions are done and the person falls over on their face, should they move the person or wait for 911?

What is Hypoxia and is it fatal?

How does a piece of plague break off in the heart causing lack of oxygen to the brain?

Could a severe argument plus high blood pressure and heart palpitations cause a person to fall over and lose consciousness?

What would cause a person in good health to keel over?

To find out the answers to these questions and learn more about this state of the art rehabilitation center and foundation: go to www.kesslerfoundation.org. Answers to many of these questions, services and evaluations can be found on their website.

Frequently Asked Questions: Elder Care Abuse

1. What is elder care abuse?
2. What are the warning signs?
3. What is self-neglect and what are the signs?
4. What makes an older adult vulnerable to abuse?
5. Who are these abusers? How can they be identified?
6. Are there criminal penalties for the abusers?
7. How many people are suffering from elder care abuse?
8. How can we make people more aware and how can I work to stop it?

True Stories

My Experiences with Care giving

Author: Barbara Ehrentreu

My experience with care giving came when my husband had a heart attack requiring by pass surgery. He was transported to Westchester Medical Center by ambulance the day after the heart attack, since the hospital where he was first taken didn't do that kind of surgery. Westchester Medical Center specialized in heart surgery. So I was very happy to see he was there. However, since he was also a patient at the Veteran's Administration the resident doctor decided to have him transferred to a Veteran's hospital facility Unfortunately, that hospital didn't do bypass surgery. When I found out about this I was angry, but I went to the ombudsman of the hospital and told them about this treatment. My husband was in an emergency need for a bypass. As soon as I saw the ombudsman and returned to my husband's room I found he was getting an X-ray and being given materials for surgery. They did the surgery the following morning and if he had waited any longer he would have died. His heart was beating at eleven per cent and his blood had turned black.

After the surgery he couldn't get off the breathing tube or wake up enough. So they left it in him for almost two weeks, which caused him to contract bacterial pneumonia. The bacterial pneumonia required the hospital to isolate my husband and we had to wear gowns and gloves when visiting him. He was not really awake and rarely communicated with us. He knew my daughters, and me but since we couldn't speak with him we had no idea what he was thinking. When he was allowed to start to talk through the tracheotomy when I was leaving he would grab my arm and say I should come early so we could talk. He did this several times and I didn't know what he was talking about until later when I needed to get his signature on a proxy form so I could pay our bills. The head of the nurses would not sign off on the paper. She said that she didn't think my husband was in his right mind. I was shocked, since he was such a logical and grounded person. So they had psychiatrists come in and interview him. Was I surprised at his answers to their questions!!! He was asked to tell them what year it was and he said 1964. Then they asked him where he was and he said he was in a Vietnamese prisoner of war camp. The diagnosis was that he had a form of delirium. Then he started to try to get out of bed all the time and the hospital had to give him one on one attendant. He would scream at them if they didn't do what he wanted and one time he got so angry with one male attendant who wouldn't give him his clothes that he kicked him. I couldn't believe that my husband did that.

I had to intervene several times during his treatment, because the VA wanted to transfer him and he wasn't ready to leave. He was given physical therapy to get him to walk better while in the hospital. Eventually, he came back to reality and returned to the logical person he had been.

Another time I had to be a caregiver was when my husband had very high calcium due to a sarcoidosis of his kidney. He was put in the hospital and given IV liquids to flush out the calcium. Then when his level was almost normal the doctors allowed him to go home and finish as an outpatient. However, the doctors prescribed both high levels of Prednisone and a new kind of insulin along with Ambien. In a few days my husband was hallucinating and then after an incident he was taken to the hospital again. There he continued to hallucinate and turned angry at night screaming at the top of his lungs and getting out of bed, though he was very unsteady. The nurses needed to restrain him, but he couldn't be contained. He was put on bed alarm, but even then it didn't help. He would rave and so he was given a drug. One night I went over to the hospital to see his behavior. While I was in his room he got out of bed and when I wouldn't get his clothes for him he slapped me. This brought the entire trauma staff to his room and he was given a large does of medicine.

Barbara Ehrentreu
If I Could Be Like Jennifer Taylor—Coming September, 2011
from MuseItUp Publishing

Barbara's Meanderings
http://barbaraehrentreu.blogspot.com/

Red River Writers Live Tales from the Pages
http://www.blogtalkradio.com/rrradio/2010/07/22/red-river-writers-live—tales-from-the-pages-with-

NY Literature Examiner for *Examiner.com*
http://www.examiner.com/x-33746-NY-Literature-Examiner-topic575176-book-reviews

DRIVING HOME

Author: Fran Lewis

My mom drove me to the doctor to one morning. Going home she made a U-Turn down a one-way street and passed three red lights and then turned down a one-way street to get home faster. When I tried to tell her she was going the wrong way she told me she knew what she was doing. At that point three police cars surrounded us. I thought I was living an episode of some cop show on television. I did not know whether to laugh or cry. When the officers approached the car and told my mom what she had done you do not want to know what she answered them: I did nothing wrong. What is your problem? Added to that she was not wearing a seatbelt and preceded to show them her scar from her heart surgery saying the belt hurt her chest. When she looked for her license and car insurance she could not find her current insurance even though it was in her wallet with her ten thousand other cards. She then told me to flirt with the officers, with a headache and feeling crappy to try and get them not to give her a ticket. By the time she got done instead of eight tickets for eight violations they let her off with a warning. It was at that point I called my sister and said it was time to take away the keys. She parked the car only to call my Aunt Tova to go to the supermarket later that day. She is a trip.

I CAN'T BREATHE!

Author: Faith McDonald

In December of 1993 my husband, David, was electrocuted and I became his caregiver as a result. As a caregiver I would like to make a suggestion to all other caregivers, if I may—BREATHE! I came to realize that David was not the only one whose life had been totally changed as a result of the electrocution, but our family as a whole was forced to go through life altering changes. You just go into performance mode. Much as do soldiers in a war and believe me, you are in a war—just a silent unknown one; not seen by many, invisible, painful and scary. You lose yourself. But, in doing so, you find yourself. I didn't know until my husband's accident that I had it within me to be a paramedic, administrator, a nurse, a paralegal, a fundraiser and a P.R. person, T.V. personality and a hero, or at least that is what our local paper referred to me as. But, those were the roles in which I found myself playing and operating. In my heart, in my mind, I was a wife, a mother and a woman that was fearful, inadequate and traumatized. It is amazing what a woman/man can be, when she or he is forced to be it in any given situation. My advice would be to take a minute (if that is all that is afforded you) light a candle, set in a quite place, without guilt, and BREATHE. Find people with whom you can talk who understand; talk therapy is essential. You can't give what you don't have. My husband's condition has much improved. He has outdone everything that the doctors said he would never do. Care giving is not a death sentence, but a rebirth into all of your and your loved ones possibilities.

Reverend Faith McDonald

Think about how many people need help and do not have family members to speak for them or take care of them. Think about how you can make a positive difference in someone's life: Volunteer: Become A Caregiver. Learn how to protect yourself, your family and your children from Traumatic Brain Injury. Protecting the Elderly is so vital and important. Learn the Causes and Signs of Eldercare Abuse and help STOP IT!

Use this book as your guide.

This book is dedicated to two of the most amazing women in my life: My sister, Marcia Wallach who died from Traumatic Brain Injury on July 8, 2010 and my mom, who made me strong, kind, responsible and caring: Ruth Swerdloff who passed away on March 7, 2010. My mom had Alzheimer's and many other heart related illnesses. She was my voice growing up and I was hers for the past 10 years. If I had to do it again I would.

Special thank you to the nurses on 9 North and 8 North in Albert Einstein Hospital in the Bronx for taking care of my mom and showing such understanding and compassion to all of your patients. To Daria Smith the nurse case manager and Anne the manager on 8 North you are so special and thank you for understanding my mom's needs and helping me when I needed your assistance.

The proceeds from this book will go for funding research to find the cause of Alzheimer's Disease. Both Montefiore Hospital & Einstein Hospital will receive necessary funds to fund their research programs and for patient care. I wrote this book because I care about the elderly and want things to change. Traumatic Brain Injury is part of the reason why I lost my sister. If I can help someone else it would be like helping her.